General Practice

Essential Facts

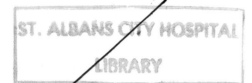

Richard Jones
and
Scott Menzies

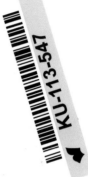

Foreword by
Roger Neighbour
Convenor, Panel of Examiners
RCGP

Radcliffe Medical Press

Radcliffe Medical Press Ltd
18 Marcham Road, Abingdon, Oxon OX14 1AA

British Library Cataloguing in Publication Data

A catalogue record for this book is available from the British Library.

ISBN 1 85775 250 3

Typeset by Multiplex Medway Ltd, Walderslade, Kent
Printed and bound by The Cromwell Press, Trowbridge, Wilts

Contents

Foreword

To practise medicine is to inhabit many parallel universes.

Those of us who work in primary care perhaps appreciate this better than our colleagues in more specialised areas of the profession. To be effective a GP must be equally at home not only in an expanding galaxy of clinical worlds but also – and this for 30 years has been the singular contribution of British general practice – in the private and privileged domain of the individual consultation. As well as honing their clinical acumen, registrars serving their apprenticeship in general practice are rightly encouraged by their trainers to sensitise themselves to the interplay of relationships within the microcosm of the consulting room.

And yet even this is not enough. There exists also a medical world beyond the surgery, a world in which clinical knowledge, though important, is not sufficient to understand why patients present in the ways *they* do and why we respond as *we* do. It makes life easier, and the job more satisfying, for us in addition to have a sense of the big picture: of how things are in the UK system of healthcare; of how things got to be the way they are; and of how intimate are the connections between the political and administrative infrastructure of the NHS on one hand and, on the other, the health inequities and moral controversies that the nation tirelessly debates.

As I write, primary care groups will shortly be upon us. They will be the latest in a long series of attempts to shield central government from being blamed when identified health needs are short-changed by inadequate resources. Now more than ever, if GPs are to be effective advocates for evidence-based health planning, we need to have demographic, historical and financial facts at our fingertips.

By providing a *vademecum* of this information Richard Jones and Scott Menzies have done the future of primary care a great service. They have pulled together an illuminating array of data which would have been impossibly daunting for the individual doctor to compile. That they have managed to do so in such a readable and stimulating style is a bonus. As an MRCGP Examiner I know to my sorrow how easy it can be for young doctors to convince themselves that ignorance of the wider context of practice, if not bliss, is at least forgivable. Thanks to this book there is no longer any excuse!

Roger Neighbour MA, FRCGP
Convenor, Panel of Examiners, RCGP
November 1998

Preface

The aim of this book is to condense the facts and figures that are available in the public domain concerning the NHS into a readable format. As trainees ourselves some years ago, we derived great benefit from the work of the late John Fry in his publications *Present State and Future Needs* and *General Practice: the facts* and we would like to acknowledge the enormous contribution that he made to general practice by producing a book in a similar vein to those previously mentioned.

We hope that this book will provide a useful source of information for candidates preparing for the MRCGP, and beyond for doctors facing the enormous challenge that a lifetime in general practice will inevitably provide. As trainers/RCGP examiners, we perceive the need for young doctors entering the profession to be able to formulate ideas and be aware of what they are letting themselves in for. As general practice is both diverse and absorbing we find it useful to sit back and reflect occasionally on what it is we actually do and to compare our subjective impressions with objective data.

As practising GPs we are all faced with multifaceted challenges which sometimes make it difficult to focus on our raison d'être. Our aim in this book is not to tell people how things should be done but rather to allow them to identify the challenges, develop their strategies for personal professional development and identify their role within the 'wider scheme of things'.

Throughout the book are areas of commentary and opinion which aim to link the facts with grass roots experience and the profession's perceptions – if your aim is to simply read the facts, these diversions should be ignored. Their aim is simply to stimulate and provoke the readers ideas and opinions.

The data: The information in this book is drawn from demographic, epidemiological, operational and clinical governmental sources found in various publications of the government health and social departments and from public health sources in our own areas of practice.

Presentation: The data are presented without elaborate statistical analysis with the aim that ordinary hard-working doctors, nurses, pharmacists, healthcare professionals and our political masters can digest them without them creating unnecessary dyspepsia or reflux.

Richard Jones
Scott Menzies
November 1998

Acknowledgements

We are extremely grateful to a great number of people who have assisted with this publication and have to apologise that all cannot be named as there are far too many to mention. However, some must be named for their unstinting efforts on our behalf; without them this would never have happened. Our thanks go to the following:

- The statisticians at the NHS Executive in Leeds. This enthusiastic group at Stats GMS, Ed Holden in particular, and many of his colleagues, never failed to deliver when the going was tough – they deserve enormous praise which I suspect is rarely attributed.
- Our partners both at home and in practice without whose tolerance and support this project would not have been completed.
- Dr Bob Mortimer who contributed at the start of this project but who suffered an unreasonable number of family medical disasters – we wish him and his family well.
- Our many colleagues in our local areas and at the RCGP who continue to stimulate us – there are some great GPs out there!
- Radcliffe Medical Press for their unhurried approach to novices like us.

1

What is general practice?

General practice in the United Kingdom provides primary care to the whole population, i.e. general practice is the main first point of contact with the National Health Service. All patients in the UK have the right of access to a general practitioner.

Roles of the GP

Demand-led care

The care provided when patients present themselves to a practice for advice or treatment. This may be provided by either the GP or by a nurse, health visitor or other health professional within the practice.

Long-term care and prevention

The management in the long term of chronic diseases, such as asthma and diabetes, where treatment according to presenting symptoms is inadequate or inappropriate. Prevention includes doctor-led surveillance and intervention to prevent or reduce illness in the long term. This may be via proactive measures such as screening programmes or 'well person' type clinics or via opportunistic methods when patients present themselves with other problems.

The business of general practice

A principal in general practice in the UK is a self-employed subcontractor within the NHS. He owns or rents the practice premises, directly employs practice staff and has control over the way the practice is run. In addition to his medical skills, he therefore requires managerial and organisational skills.

A primary care-led NHS

General practitioners in the UK have always played an important role in safeguarding the NHS, particularly with regard to controlling access to secondary care. The influence of GPs expanded significantly with the introduction of the 1990 Contract and the advent of fundholding and commissioning of care. Since 1990 there has been far more emphasis on the needs of primary care and GPs have been instrumental in guiding the development of secondary services and the way they are provided. This is reflected in the term 'primary care-led NHS', which reflects the government's aims for further development in the health service. The role of the GP is likely to become even more important over the next decade.

The hierarchy of healthcare provision

Common to all systems of healthcare are various levels of care ranging from self-care in the home to superspecialist care in national centres.

Self-care

Most episodes of illness are managed by the sufferers themselves, often with the assistance of immediate family. This has traditionally been augmented with help from extended family, such as grandparents, whose role has been eroded over recent decades with changes in the structure of society and the breakdown of the nuclear family. This clearly has implications for the health service.

Primary care

In the UK, general practice provides the first level of professional care, accessed when self-care is deemed inadequate. General practices are based within the population they cover and an average practice will provide care for up to about 20 000 patients.

General specialist care

District general hospitals cover populations up to about 500 000 and provide the first level of secondary care. Services include general medicine and surgery, paediatrics, obstetrics, gynaecology, accident and emergency, orthopaedics and generally ear, nose and throat surgery and ophthalmology. With the exception of accident and emergency and sexually transmitted diseases, patients do not generally have direct access to specialist care via self-referral.

Superspecialist care

Regional centres provide care for larger populations of up to 5 million. These house superspecialist care, such as cardiothoracic surgery, plastic surgery, neurosurgery, etc. Referral can be either from general specialists in district general hospitals or from GPs.

Thus, as we move from the level of self-care towards superspecialist care, the numbers involved increase, as does the level of specialism. Around three-quarters of problems are managed by self-care and of those taken to the GP, around nine-tenths are managed within primary care.

Each level of care has its own:

- roles, functions and limitations
- content of morbidity and problems
- skills, tools, methods and resources
- training, teaching and learning needs
- research, audit and monitoring.

This book will focus on the above features which relate to general practice in the UK.

Features of British general practice

- Single route of access to the NHS except for accident and emergency and genitourinary clinics.
- Direct access to 24-hour care.
- Comprehensive first-contact care involving diagnosis, investigation and treatment.
- Co-ordination of local medical and social services for individual patients and families.
- Gatekeeping and protection of local hospitals through the selective referral process.
- Relatively small and stable population bases of about 1700 patients per GP, often in groups, for example five GPs and 8500 patients.
- Long-term generalist, personal and family care within the community, by doctors and primary healthcare team, of patients who often come to know each other well over the years.
- The content in terms of morbidity and mortality will correspond to the size of practice (see Chapters 2 and 4).
- The GP has the central role for provision of good health within the local community.

Figure 1.1 Flow of care.

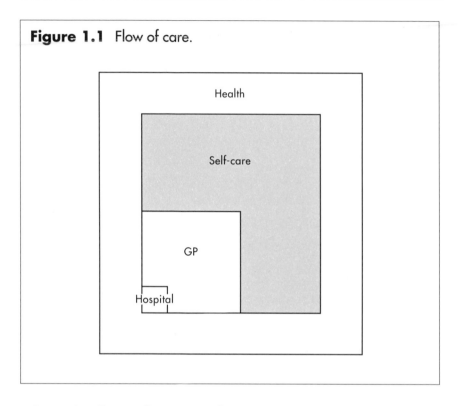

Historical evolution of British general practice

The first references to a 'general medical practitioner' appeared about 200 years ago. The development of general practice as a specialist field and of its status has been slow. Some notable key events are:

1815	Apothecaries Act recognised the Surgeon-Apothecary and the Society of Apothecaries (GPs)
1841	Royal Pharmaceutical Society of Great Britain (RPSGB) set up
1858	General Medical Council (GMC) set up to control standards and conduct, educate doctors and to protect the public and profession from quacks and lay healers

1911	David Lloyd George's National Health Insurance Act, providing compulsory prepaid health and medical insurance for employees below certain agreed low wages
1914	First World War
1920	Dawson Report setting out the future concept of health centres and primary and secondary care
1939	Second World War
1942	Beveridge Report on setting up the Welfare State
1948	National Health Service set up under Labour government with Aneurin Bevan as Minister of Health (amidst reluctance from GPs)
1952	College of General Practitioners founded (amidst reluctance from specialists)
1966	Charter for General Practice, by government and profession, creating inducements with staff reimbursements, rent/rates reimbursements, seniority awards, higher rates of pay and items of service, pay for continuing education and for group practices (over three partners)
1982	Compulsory three-year vocational training for GP principals
1990	New Contract for general practice with emphasis on better value for NHS money, audit, practice reports and leaflets, targets for immunisation and cervical cytology, attempted control of prescribing, hospital referrals, staff employment and budget holdings
1997	Summative assessment made compulsory for all registrars
1998	Development of primary care groups to replace fundholding

Discussion

1 General practice is the essential base level in all health systems, with its own roles, functions, features and tools.
2 General practice within the NHS provides direct, available and accessible care to a small and stable community over many years.
3 Historical evolution of general practice in the UK since 1815 has created a stable system of primary healthcare that is the envy of the world.

2

UK demography

Population

The population of the UK was approximately 58.4 million in 1996 and is projected to rise by another million by 2001. There was a 3% increase between 1983 and 1993 overall but, perhaps more significantly, the percentage of over 65-year-olds has risen by 9% and the percentage of over 75-year-olds has risen by 13% in the same period.

Table 2.1 UK population by age

	<5	5–14	15–29	30–44	45–64	65–74	75–84	85+	Total
No. of persons (millions)	3.9	7.5	12.3	12.5	13.0	5.1	3.1	1.0	58.4
% of total population	6.7	12.8	21.1	21.4	22.3	8.7	5.3	1.7	100

(Source: OHE Compendium of Health Statistics, 1995)

Table 2.2 Male:female ratios in the UK

Country	Male (millions)	Female (millions)	Total (millions)	Male %	Female %
England and Wales	25.28	26.32	51.6	43.3	45.09
Scotland	2.49	2.65	5.14	4.26	4.54
Northern Ireland	0.8	0.83	1.63	1.37	1.44
Total	28.57	29.8	58.37	48.93	51.07

Figure 2.1 UK population – age distribution.

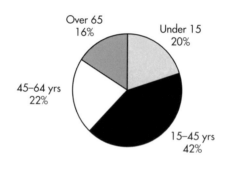

Figure 2.2 UK population by country and percentage.

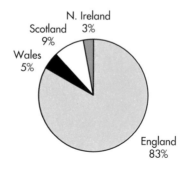

Elderly population

The percentage of persons in the UK overall aged 65 years or over was 15.6% in 1995 and there was a 9% increase between 1983 and 1993. The over 75-year-olds comprised 6.7% of the total population in 1995, with a 13% increase between 1983 and 1993.

Life expectancy

The life expectancy (at birth) in the UK has almost doubled over the past 150 years. Babies born in 1996 can expect to live in excess of 70 years with males averaging 74.5 years and females 78.8 years. See Table 2.3 to compare life expectancy for both sexes in 1841!

Table 2.3 Life expectancy 1841–1996

Year	1841	1901	1920	1948	1960	1970	1980	1990	1996 (Estimate)
Male	40.2	48.5	55.6	66.4	68.3	68.8	70.4	73.2	74.5
Female	42.2	52.4	59.6	71.2	74.1	75.1	76.6	78.7	79.8

(Source: OHE Compendium of Health Statistics, 1995)

Table 2.4 shows how we compare with other developed countries.

Table 2.4 International life expectancy at birth in OECD countries 1995–2000 (projections)

Country	Male	Female
World average	59.5	63.3
Western Europe average	70.7	77.7
EEC average	71.1	77.5

Table 2.4 Cont'd

Country	Male	Female
UK	71.0	77.2
USA	70.9	78.3
Australia	71.9	78.7
Canada	72.4	79.6
France	70.8	78.9
Germany	70.3	76.8
Japan	74.2	79.7
Turkey	60.0	64.6

(Source: World Population Prospects, United Nations, 1992)

Births

The birth rate in the UK is now almost one-third of the rate 120 years ago but, perhaps more importantly, the infant death rate (which is expressed as deaths under one year of age) has been reduced 25-fold. The UK infant death rate has decreased by 42% in the ten-year period 1983–1993.

Table 2.5 Trends in birth and infant death rates 1870–1993

Year	1870	1900	1920	1940	1960	1970	1980	1990	1993
Live births per 1000 population	35.0	28.6	23.1	14.6	17.5	16.3	13.5	13.9	13.1
Infant deaths per 1000 live births	149.7	142.5	81.9	61.0	22.5	18.5	12.1	7.9	5.9

(Source: Annual Abstracts of Statistics and OPCS)

Deaths

The crude death rate (includes all deaths and all ages) was 10.9 per 1000 population in 1993 compared with 22.1 in 1870. The crude death rate dropped by 6% between 1983 and 1993. There were 631 287 deaths in 1992, of which 549 998 were from natural causes.

The main causes of death were:

- circulatory 47%
- cancer 27%
- respiratory 11%
- other 15%

The trend has been for circulatory and respiratory deaths to decrease over the last 25 years whereas cancer deaths have stayed at approximately the same level.

Families

The average number of births to women during their reproductive years was 1.8 in 1993 and the trend has been towards smaller families over the past 25 years. Clearly if this figure stays below 2.0, then the population will drop below the present level.

Table 2.6 Trends in family size 1951–93

Year	1951	1961	1971	1981	1991	1993
Average births per woman	2.15	2.80	2.41	1.81	1.90	1.80

(Sources: Social Trends and private communication Dr J Whittington)

Of all births, 31.8% were illegitimate according to census definitions, i.e. born out of wedlock, which represents a massive rise compared to the figure of 5% which was static until 1960.

In 1993 the marriage rate was 6.1 per 1000 population and the divorce rate was 3.0 per 1000 population. This is clearly of concern since the marriage:divorce ratio of 49.2% represents a large degree of change compared to the 41.3% figure quoted for 1987.

Discussion

1 The population of the UK is 58.4 million and has risen by 3% in a decade despite increased availability of reliable forms of contraception.

2 Life expectancy has almost doubled over the past 150 years and of more relevance perhaps is that the geriatric population is rising markedly with a 9% increase in the last decade. The over-75s have increased by 13% in the past decade. This will have an enormous implication in terms of health resource management and GP workload statistics.

3 Birth rates are relatively low and are less than the two babies per woman required to maintain the population; therefore, the overall figure must be rising due to immigration.

4 Infant deaths are at an all-time low, there being only 5.9 per 1000 live births.

5 Almost 1:2 marriages ends in divorce, which is a marked rise on previously quoted figures. This creates considerable social morbidity and has implications for the workload of GPs and allied health and social sector workers.

6 Almost every third child is born to an unmarried mother.

7 Circulatory diseases still account for almost 50% of all deaths. Despite considerable work in this area, we as a profession are not significantly altering this fact. Consider what needs to be done to make an impact on this.

3

The NHS

Historical review

The NHS was set up in 1948. The main events which have influenced the evolution of general practice along the way are as follows.

- 1950   Collings Report
- 1952   College of General Practitioners formed
- 1963   Gillie Report (health team)
- 1965/6 Charter for General Practice
- 1974   Family practitioner committees (FPCs) set up
- 1980   United Kingdom Central Council (UKCC) set up for nurses, midwives and health visitors
- 1982   Vocational training introduced for GPs
- 1985   FPCs become more independent
- 1990   New Contract
- 1991   NHS and Community Care Act
- 1992   *Health of the Nation* published – standards and targets
- 1998   *Our Healthier Nation* published

Structure of the NHS in England

The administrative system of the NHS in the UK is based on a hierarchical structure, though current government policy is to allow more autonomy and to move towards local decision making within central guidelines.

The head of the NHS in England is the Secretary of State for Health, based within the Department of Health (DoH). In Wales, Scotland and Northern Ireland it is the Secretary of State for each country. All are answerable to Parliament. The role of the DoH in England is to formulate health policy, advise ministers, deal with public health issues and instruct the NHS Executive headquarters (the head office of the NHS).

The 1989 White Paper *Working for Patients* created the concept of 'purchasers' and 'providers' of healthcare. District health authorities (DHAs) were to evolve into purchasing agencies. NHS hospitals could either become NHS trusts outside DHA control or remain within the NHS structure as directly managed units (DMUs). Larger general practices were to be offered the chance to become fund-holders, purchasing certain services directly on behalf of their patients. These changes came into being in April 1991 following the *NHS and Community Care Act 1990*.

Further evolution occurred and in April 1996, regional health authorities (RHAs) were abolished and district health authorities and family health service authorities merged to form 100 health authorities following the *Health Authorities Act 1995*.

Secretary of State

The head of the NHS in England is the Secretary of State for Health. He or she chairs the NHS Policy Board which is responsible for a number of strategic and financial issues, licensing new drugs and setting official health targets. The board is accountable to Parliament and a number of parliamentary committees.

NHS Executive

The NHS Executive is the administrative head office of the NHS in England. It is run by a chief executive who is accountable to ministers. Since April 1996 the NHS Executive has monitored the provision of healthcare through eight regional offices, taking over the role previously undertaken by RHAs and Outpost offices, providing a link between strategic and local management. These regions are Anglia and Oxford, North Thames, South Thames, South and West, West Midlands, North West, Northern and Yorkshire, and Trent. Each is headed by a regional director.

Purchasers of healthcare

Purchasers of healthcare are free to negotiate contracts with both NHS and non-NHS providers.

Following the formation of 100 health authorities in 1996, the purchase of healthcare is done by each authority at a local level, while still having a responsibility to implement national policy. The names may vary (e.g. health agency, health commission) but the function still remains the same. They are responsible for managing terms of service for GPs, dentists, opticians and pharmacists as well as monitoring the quality of healthcare services agreed in contracts. They have a role in developing primary care and in overseeing patient registration with GPs.

With the advent of locality purchasing and the formation of primary care commissioning groups to replace GP fundholding, these authorities are increasingly involving GPs in the decision-making process and a number of different models are evolving, giving primary care an important role in shaping local policies.

Providers of healthcare

Independent contractors

GPs, dentists, pharmacists and opticians are independent contractors within the NHS under contracts negotiated by the Department of Health. These contracts are administered by the local health authority.

NHS trusts

NHS trusts are self-governing public corporations within the NHS. The board of each trust consists of a chairman, five executive directors and five non-executive directors. The trusts can provide a full range of health services or specialise in activities such as community health services, mental health services or ambulance services.

In 1991–92, 96% of the core income for first-wave NHS trusts came from DHAs. Trusts provide more than 90% of all NHS secondary healthcare services.

Directly managed units

Directly managed units are healthcare providers which have not become NHS trusts and are under the administration of the local health authority.

Management levels

Management of the NHS may be related to population levels as shown in Figure 3.1.

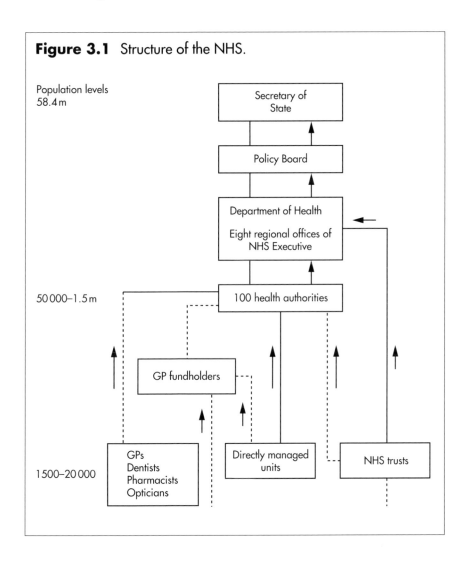

Figure 3.1 Structure of the NHS.

Population levels
58.4 m

Secretary of State

Policy Board

Department of Health

Eight regional offices of NHS Executive

50 000–1.5 m   100 health authorities

GP fundholders

1500–20 000   GPs / Dentists / Pharmacists / Opticians

Directly managed units

NHS trusts

Parliament is responsible for the entire NHS in the UK.

General practices are independent and under contract to the health authorities.

Families manage approximately 75% of all health problems themselves.

Health Authorities. This is the management level between the DoH and the providers of health including responsibility for district general hospitals, general practice, dentists, pharmacists and opticians.

Department of Health. There is one for each of the home nations, headed by a Chief Medical Officer.

NHS staff

The NHS is the largest civilian employer in Europe and employs approximately 1 million people or approximately one in 40 workers.

Table 3.1 NHS staff	
Occupation	%
Nurses	50
Doctors (hospital)	5.7
GPs	3.2
Professional/technical	11.3
Managers/administrators	18.6
Domestic, maintenance, ambulance and transport, etc.	11.2
(Source: OHE Compendium of Health Statistics, 1995)	

Figure 3.2 NHS hospital manpower per 100 000 population, UK Index 1951 = 100. (Source: *Compendium of Health Statistics, 1995*.)

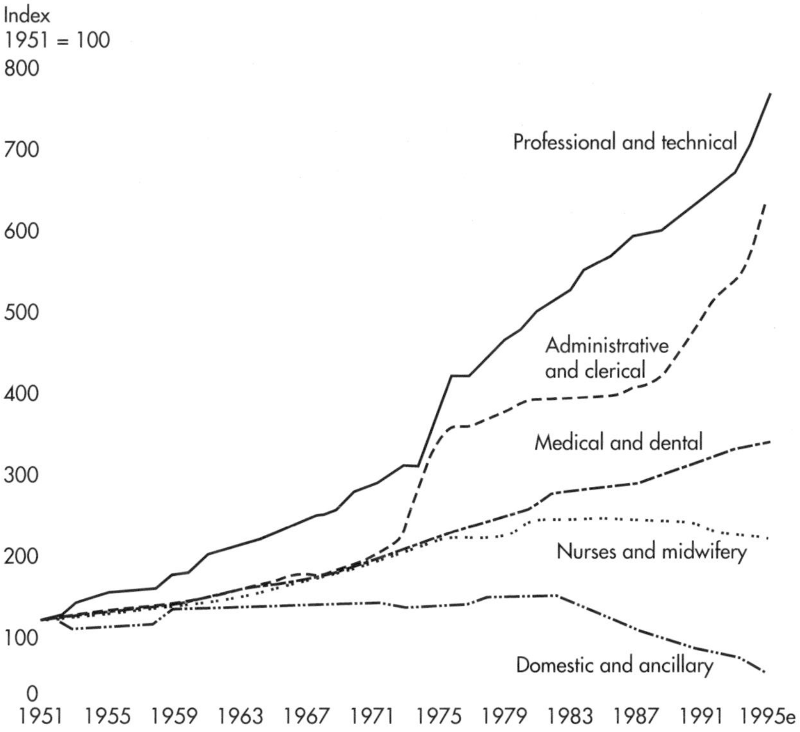
Index
1951 = 100
800
700
600
500
400
300
200
100
0
1951 1955 1959 1963 1967 1971 1975 1979 1983 1987 1991 1995e
Professional and technical
Administrative and clerical
Medical and dental
Nurses and midwifery
Domestic and ancillary

Discussion

1 There have been vast changes in the NHS in the past decade and that process of change looks set to continue into the next millennium. What audit(s) has been performed to evaluate the effects on patients and healthcare professionals?
2 Data pertaining to healthcare needs within the NHS exist. How effective are we as a profession in predicting future needs across all strata of society?

4

The content of practice

Since general practice is the first level of primary professional care, the activities and content reflect both first-contact care and the morbidity and mortality of small but relatively stable population bases. Data collected from general practice estimate the incidence and prevalence of disease seen at this level.

Definitions

The **incidence** of a disease is taken to be the number of new episodes of a condition or group of conditions diagnosed during the study year, i.e. the sum of first ever (F) and new (N) episodes reported.

The **prevalence** of a disease is the level of presence of a disease during the study year and is defined as the number of persons who consulted at least once for a condition or group of conditions during the year. Incidence and prevalence are shown in the tables below as rates per 10 000 person-years at risk.

Please note that it is possible for an individual to contribute once to the prevalence of a disease, but several times to the incidence of that disease if he has experienced more than one distinct episode of that disease during the year.

These data can give us an insight into the demand made on the health service at the main point of entry and so hopefully help us plan to meet this need. Most of the data that follow in this chapter are taken from the Fourth National Study (1991–92) into Morbidity Statistics from General Practice, in which more detailed analysis can be found.

Severity of illness

Most illnesses are minor, self-limiting and short-lived and so the GP tends to see a preponderance of these; however, major life-threatening illness and disabling diseases present in approximately 15% of GP consultations. Whilst being less prevalent, they are often more demanding in terms of the care required. The middle group of disorders, classed intermediate, include many chronic disorders the proportion of which is shown in Figure 4.1. Although the majority of consultations are for minor and intermediate conditions, it would be wrong to assume that GPs represent a cadre of lower-grade doctors; quite the opposite as the problems require just as much skilled care and careful consideration as do the more serious, major conditions.

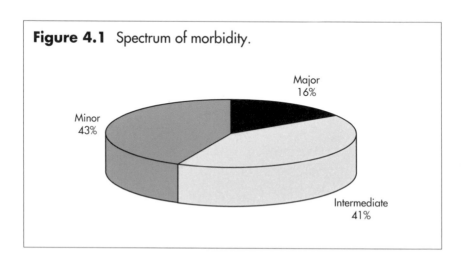

Figure 4.1 Spectrum of morbidity.

The spectrum of disease and sickness that presents in general practice is more representative than that in a hospital setting because those patients attending hospital are preselected for referral by GPs, except in the case of accident and emergency care, sexually transmitted diseases and dental care. Hence, the GP has a role as *gatekeeper* to the secondary and further care services.

Population demography

As a rough guide each GP will have 2000 patients registered on his or her list and the majority of GPs (70%) work in groups. However, depending upon location of the practice and other social factors, each practice profile can differ quite markedly. Tables 4.1 and 4.2 show the profiles for the authors' practices, which serve very different populations, resulting in differing workloads.

Table 4.1 Practice 1 – Langford Medical Practice 10.8.97

Age	0–4	5–14	15–29	30–44	45–64	65–74	75–84	85+
Male	459	630	790	1302	453	69	23	5
% age cf UK average	187%	137%	80%	152%	58%	24%	16%	15%
Female	436	616	1093	1437	446	63	36	6
% age cf UK average	186%	142%	115%	169%	56%	17%	14%	8%

Table 4.2 Practice 2 – Kingsway Swansea Medical Practice 9.9.97

Age	0–4	5–14	15–29	30–44	45–64	65–74	75–84	85+
Male	279	590	984	941	943	355	148	25
% age cf UK average	102%	115%	90%	99%	108%	110%	92%	67%
Female	273	561	994	905	1013	409	265	97
% age cf UK average	104%	116%	94%	95%	114%	99%	92%	116%

Implications for workload

Births

The present birth rate is 13.1 per 1000 so that Practice 1 might expect about 96 births in a 12-month period; however, in 1996–97 there were 178 confinements. This could be predicted from the very high proportion of female patients of childbearing age compared to national figures. Clearly, the geriatric population in Practice 2 forms a much higher proportion of the total than Practice 1 and so provision for this workload needs careful planning. Thus, an understanding of population statistics relevant to one's own practice can allow suitable provision of care to be tailored towards the expected needs of the patients.

Deaths

The annual crude death rate is 10.9 per 1000, so there will be 22 deaths per GP with 2000 patients. Practice 1 might have expected 80 deaths in 1996–97 but in fact there were only 11. Study of the practice demography again might be thought to influence this result.

Figure 4.2 Place of death.

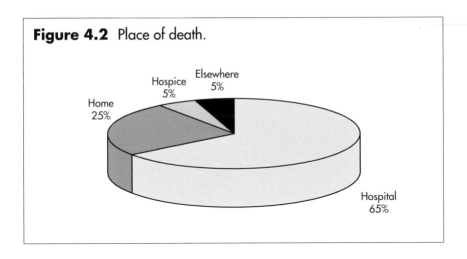

Table 4.3 Leading causes of deaths (male and female per 100 000 population UK)

Total deaths	1506
From natural causes	948
Ischaemic heart disease	259
Cerebrovascular disease	117
Malignant disease	109
Pneumonia	48
Diabetes mellitus	14
Bronchitis/emphysema	11

(Source: OHE Compendium of Health Statistics, 1992)

Clinical content of consultations

One of the purposes of this book is to identify changes in morbidity seen in general practice and thus the results of the 1981–82 National Morbidity Study and the 1991–92 Study have been compared. The figures quoted are those of prevalence, which for these purposes is defined as the number of persons consulting at least once during the study year expressed as a rate per 10 000 person-years at risk. This

may be lengthened by earlier diagnosis or as the result of treatment. An example is cancer of the breast. The prevalence rate increased between 1981–82 and 1991–92, but the first incidence rate remained the same, suggesting that the chance of developing cancer of the breast is unchanged but the average survival has increased.

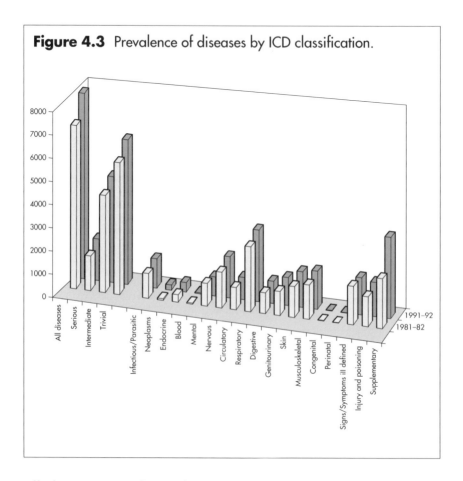

Figure 4.3 Prevalence of diseases by ICD classification.

All diseases and conditions

The graph in Figure 4.3 shows the changes in prevalence rates between 1981–82 and 1991–92 for all conditions and diseases and for each ICD chapter. Between the 1981–82 and 1991–92 surveys there was an increase from 71% to 78% in the proportion of people who consulted at least once during the study year for any disease or condition. Clearly this has implications in terms of health planning at both practice and health authority levels. The increase was greatest among the elderly, but occurred among people in every age group and both sexes.

There was an increase in the proportion of people within each age group who consulted for serious, for intermediate and for trivial conditions. Patient consulting rates increased between 1981–82 and 1991–92 for conditions in every ICD chapter except mental disorders and the chapter entitled symptoms, signs and ill-defined conditions.

The number of consultations increased by 2.4% from 33 961 per 100 000 person-years at risk in 1981–82 to 34 785 in 1991–92.

Table 4.4 shows prevalence rates for common chronic conditions and again is included to demonstrate how knowledge of these data can assist in health service provision.

Table 4.4 Prevalence rates for common chronic conditions

	1981–82	1991–92	Percentage change
CVS diseases			
Hypertension	741	806	+8.7
Acute MI	87	58	−33.3
Angina	139	228	+64
Cerebrovascular disease	82	131	+59.8
Endocrine			
Thyroid disease	91	117	+28.6
Diabetes	147	221	+50.3
Respiratory			
Asthma	359	851	+137
Chronic bronchitis	121	91	−24.8
Digestive system	1436	1751	+21.9
Selected CNS/sensory			
Migraine	160	227	+41.9
Cataract	22	34	+54.5
Glaucoma	12	21	+75
Conjunctivitis	284	396	+39.4

(Source: OPCS Morbidity Statistics from GP Fourth National Study, 1991–92)

Table 4.5 Consulting rates for generalised conditions

ICD group	Persons consulting GP per annum
Respiratory	600
Nervous/sense organ disease	340
Dermatological	300
Musculoskeletal	300
Gastrointestinal	180
Genitourinary	220
Injury/poisoning	280
Infectious and parasitic	280
Symptoms, signs and ill defined	300

Upper respiratory infections are the most prevalent cause of illness in all developed countries.

Malignant disease

Cancer is a distressing condition for both patients and doctors and there has been a 77% increase in the prevalence of 'all cancers' in the past decade. It is important to understand the workload implications which can be disproportionate to the actual prevalence of the condition. Each GP is likely to deal with about 14 new cancers per 2000 patients per year.

In the UK during 1991 (the most recent year for which UK incidence figures are available) over 273 000 people were registered with a malignant neoplasm, i.e. nearly 750 new cases every day. From such statistics, it is estimated that one in three people is at risk of developing cancer at some time during their life. However, it is likely to be later in life, with >70% of all new cases being diagnosed in people over 60 years of age.

Table 4.6 The ten commonest cancers in men and women

Number	Male %	Female %	Number
28 420	Lung 21	Breast 25	34 590
16 930	Skin* 13	Skin* 11	15 390
15 550	Prostate 12	Lung 10	13 760
9260	Bladder 7	Colon 8	10 730
9220	Colon 7	Ovary 4	5940
6920	Stomach 5	Rectum 4	4990
6510	Rectum 5	Stomach 3	4480
3890	NHL** 3	Cervix 3	4340
3540	Oesophagus 3	Uterus 3	4210
3410	Pancreas 3	Bladder 3	3650
135 040 Total	100 ∞	100 ∞	138 090 Total

(Source: CRC Scientific Report 1996–97)

* = Non-melanoma skin cancer; **NHL = Non-Hodgkin's lymphoma ∞ = Excludes benign and in situ neoplasms and those of uncertain behaviour and unspecified nature.

Prevalence

It is estimated that the number of people with a history of cancer who are alive at any given time amounts to 1% of the population, i.e. approximately 500 000 people in England and Wales and around 70 000 in Scotland.

Survival

Survival from cancer varies enormously, depending upon the type and the stage at which it is diagnosed. The five-year survival rates for some of the commonest cancers are shown in Figures 4.4 and 4.5.

Figure 4.4 Five-year relative survival (male).

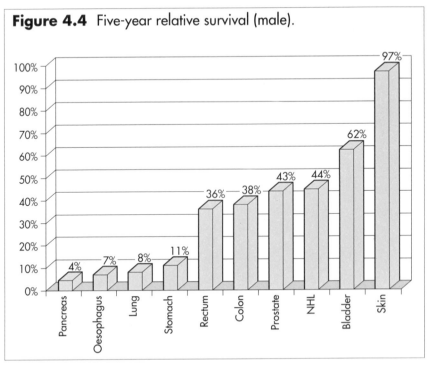

Figure 4.5 Five-year relative survival (female).

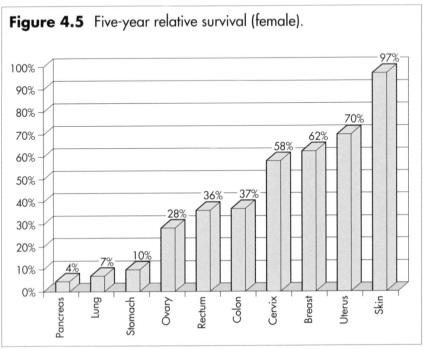

Cancer mortality

The latest available mortality statistics for the UK are for deaths occurring in 1995. However, when comparing these data to previous sets, they should be interpreted with caution due to the introduction of a new method of coding cause of death in England and Wales.

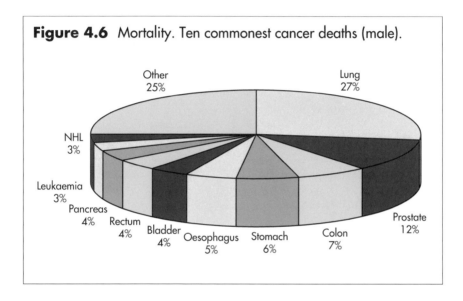

Figure 4.6 Mortality. Ten commonest cancer deaths (male).

Male – All cancers = 83 150 = 100%

One-third of all male cancer deaths are from lung cancer which is overwhelmingly due to cigarette smoking. This is also the second biggest cancer threat to women, responsible for one-sixth of all female cancer deaths. In Scotland, lung cancer has overtaken breast cancer to become the commonest cause of female cancer death.

Figure 4.7 Mortality. Ten commonest cancer deaths (female).

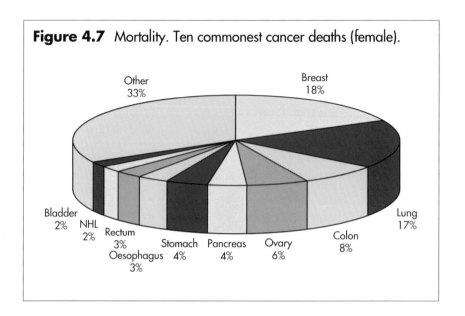

Preventive activities

More patients consulted under this ICD classification than in any other single category. This group included those patients consulting for factors influencing their health status and other contacts with the health services. Fourteen percent of the total population attended in the study year for vaccination and other preventive procedures against communicable disease.

Of women aged 16–24 and 25–44 years, 47% and 26% respectively visited their practices for contraceptive management. Among children under five years, 18% were seen for health supervision which included routine health checks.

Five percent of people visited their practices for administrative purposes, such as the issue of medical certificates, and medical examinations for expert advice, such as those requested by insurance companies.

Nearly all who attended for screening examinations for neoplasms were women; the majority of these were for screening for cervical neoplasia.

Many of the preventive tasks can be more than adequately performed by appropriately trained health professionals other than GPs. Delegation of much of this activity, much of which is remunerated separately to GMS since the 1990 Contract, has allowed GPs to cope with the massive increase in preventive workload. It is estimated that 25% of a GP's workload is involved with preventive procedures.

Discussion

1 It is important to understand the difference between the incidence and the prevalence of diseases in order to plan appropriately for future health needs.

2 Most episodes of illness seen by GPs are minor, self-limiting and short-lived. Should there be a role for other health professionals, e.g. nurse practitioners, in dealing with this area of work?

3 Fifteen percent of GP consultations are for major life-threatening and disabling diseases so the GP's role in sorting the wheat from the chaff should never be underestimated.

4 Each GP has approximately 2000 patients registered and 70% work in groups, which allows some economy of scale.

5 Population demography can influence workload dramatically and specific areas of work particularly.

6 In the 1991–92 Morbidity Study 78% of patients consulted at least once during the study year.

7 There was an increase in the proportion of people within each age group who consulted for serious, intermediate and minor conditions. Patient consulting rates increased between 1981–82 and 1991–92 for conditions in every ICD chapter other than mental disorders and symptoms, signs and ill-defined conditions.

8 It is estimated that the number of people with a history of cancer who are alive at any given time amounts to 1% of the population.
9 There has been a 77% increase in the prevalence of 'all cancers' in the past decade.
10 One in three people is at risk of developing cancer at some time during their life.
11 Twenty-three percent of GP workload results from preventive care. How should this be most appropriately organised?

5

General practitioners

General practitioner principals form the largest group of senior doctors in the NHS. There are approximately 34 000 in the UK, with recent figures for England and Wales demonstrating that there has been a rise of 11% in the number of unrestricted principals from 24 035 in 1985 to 26 702 in 1995. The rate of growth in their numbers has exceeded the population growth in the same period so that there were about 54.6 unrestricted principals per 100 000 population in 1995 compared to 50.9 in 1985.

Definitions

An *unrestricted principal* is a practitioner who provides the full range of general medical services (GMS) and whose list is not limited to any particular group of persons. In a few cases he or she may be relieved of the liability to have patients assigned to him or her or for emergency calls out of hours from patients other than his or her own.

A *restricted principal* is a practitioner who either:

- provides the full range of GMS but whose list is limited to the staff of one or more hospitals or similar institutions in which he or she is employed or to patients resident in or connected with one or more schools or other institutions or establishments or
- provides maternity medical services and/or contraceptive services only.

An *assistant* is a practitioner who acts as an assistant to a principal.

A *registrar* is a practitioner employed for a period of usually one year for the purposes of training in general practice and in respect of whom a training grant is paid.

Table 5.1 General practitioners by status and sex, England and Wales 1996

	All practitioners	Unrestricted principals	Restricted principals	Assistants	Registrars
England	20 010M : 8978F	19 056M : 7774F	65M : 52F	249M : 413F	640M : 740F
Percent	69 : 31	71 : 29	56 : 44	38 : 62	46 : 54
Wales	1352M : 498F	1299M : 427F	1M : 2F	11M : 16F	41M : 53F

Table 5.2 General practitioners by status and sex 1985–95 (England)

	1985	1986	1987	1988	1989	1990	1991	1992	1993	1994	1995	% age change
All practitioners	26 190	26 529	27 023	27 420	27 749	27 523	27 888	28 185	28 460	28 736	28 869	10.2
Unrestricted principals	24 035	24 460	24 922	25 322	25 608	25 622	25 686	25 968	26 289	26 567	26 702	11.1
Restricted principals	169	161	160	159	164	149	138	138	147	142	127	–24.9
Assistants	228	254	231	254	242	190	425	466	495	581	636	178.9
Trainees / Registrar	1758	1654	1710	1685	1735	1562	1639	1613	1529	1445	1404	–20.1

Table 5.2 Cont'd

Males												
All practitioners	20 714	20 777	20 901	20 915	20 863	20 519	20 364	20 332	20 243	20 179	20 007	−3.4
Unrestricted principals	19 473	19 593	19 718	19 792	19 778	19 529	19 256	19 236	19 252	19 218	19 092	−2.0
Restricted principals	101	100	101	100	103	95	82	81	87	82	73	−27.7
Assistants	99	107	100	98	91	77	174	186	200	227	237	139.4
Trainees / Registrars	1041	977	982	925	891	818	852	829	704	652	605	−41.9
Females												
All practitioners	5476	5752	6122	6505	6886	7004	7524	7853	8217	8557	8862	61.8
Unrestricted principals	4562	4867	5204	5530	5830	6093	6430	6732	7037	7349	7610	66.8
Restricted principal	68	61	59	59	61	54	56	57	60	60	54	−20.6
Assistants	129	147	131	156	151	113	251	280	295	354	399	209.3
Trainees / Registrars	717	677	728	760	844	744	787	784	825	793	799	11.4
Unrestricted principals per 100 000 population	50.9	51.7	52.5	53.2	53.6	53.4	53.3	53.7	54.2	54.5	54.6	

There has been a considerable increase in the number of female doctors during the past decade. In 1985, 19% were female whereas ten years later, they represented 28% of the total. Clearly this has implications in terms of planning for provision of care for the current and next decade should the trend continue, as it appears to indicate that it will.

The new Contract for GPs, introduced in 1990, provided for more flexible working arrangements, introducing job sharing and formalising part-time commitment. The majority (88%) of doctors were contracted to work full time in 1995, i.e. available to patients for at least 26 hours per week. Almost a third of female doctors were either job sharing or had part-time availability commitment to their patients (Table 5.3).

A retirement age of 70 years for GPs was introduced from April 1991 and there are now no doctors aged 70 or over. Over the last decade, the proportion of doctors under 30 years has fallen by over 2%, whereas the number of doctors aged over 60 years has dropped by over 6%.

Table 5.3 Contractual commitment of doctors by sex 1990–95

	1990	1991	1992	1993	1994	1995
Total (number)	25 622	25 686	25 968	26 289	26 567	26 702
Full time %	94.5	92.9	91.7	90.3	88.8	87.6
Job share %	1.0	1.5	1.8	2.0	2.3	2.4
Half time %	0.9	1.5	2.2	2.9	3.6	4.3
$^3/_4$ time %	3.5	4.0	4.4	4.8	5.3	5.7
Males (number)	19 529	19 256	19 236	19 252	19 218	19 092
Full time %	97.7	97.5	97.2	96.5	95.8	95.3
Job share %	0.5	0.7	0.7	0.8	1.0	1.1
Half time %	0.5	0.6	0.9	1.3	1.6	1.9
$^3/_4$ time %	1.3	1.2	1.2	1.4	1.6	1.6
Females (number)	6093	6430	6732	7037	7349	7610
Full time %	94.4	79.4	75.9	73.3	70.5	68.4
Job share %	2.7	3.8	4.8	5.2	5.6	5.7
Half time %	2.1	4.2	5.9	7.3	9.0	10.1
$^3/_4$ time %	0.8	12.5	13.4	14.2	14.9	15.8

Doctors and the population

The number of doctors in England rose by 11% between 1985 and 1995 from 24 035 to 26 702. The rate of growth in their numbers has been faster than the population growth, so that by 1995 there were about 54.6 doctors per 100 000 population compared with 50.9 in 1985. This does not mean, however, that their job has become relatively easier as a number of other factors have been responsible for increasing the workload in other ways.

List sizes

In the NHS, patients register with the doctor of their choice for care to be provided to them. Each GP is paid by capitation fees (i.e. per patient registered with him or her) and from other contractual payments for items of service. Therefore, it is important for GPs and managers to understand the implications of list sizes upon GPs.

Table 5.4 shows how list sizes have changed over the last 45 years.

Table 5.4 Mean list sizes per NHS principal 1950–95

	1950	1960	1970	1980	1985	1990	1995
Average list size	2500	2257	2413	2189	2068	1942	1887

(Sources: Fry J and DOH Statistical Bulletin, 1985–95)

There are slight national variations in these figures, Table 5.4 representing England. Recently released figures for 1996 show the average list size in England to be 1882 and in Wales to be 1719. Additionally, there are regional variations within each country with, for example, North Thames having an average list size of 2006 patients whereas the South and West region has only 1712 patients per GP.

The age of GPs

The average age of the GP is going down. More young doctors are becoming principals and since 1990, when the maximum age for retirement in the NHS became 70 years, the number of older doctors has decreased. The proportion of GPs under 50 years of age has risen from 58% in 1979 to 72% in 1996 (source: GMS Statistics 1996). This has an implication on career length, as Table 5.5 indicates that only 1% of doctors are under 30 years old and only 28% over 50 years old. Therefore, the vast majority are in the 30–50 year age band.

Table 5.5 Age variations of unrestricted principals (n = 26 830)

Age	<30	30–34	35–39	40–44	45–49	50–54	55–59	60–64	65-69
Number	384	3763	5416	4858	4714	3537	2463	1298	397
Percent	1	14	20	18	18	13	9	5	1

Place of birth

In the UK, 25% of GP principals were born and qualified overseas. Many overseas doctors came to the UK in the 1970s and 1980s, a large proportion from the Indian subcontinent. They represent a cohort of GPs now aged between 45 and 65 years and so replacements for their positions may well have to be found in the next few years. The 1990s have seen an increase in the number of EEC trainees/registrars arriving in the UK for the purposes of vocational training and it is therefore likely that some of these will decide to settle and become principals in the future.

Table 5.6 GP principals – place of birth

Country	1976 (%)	1989 (%)	1996 (%)
UK	74.8	74.1	82.2
Indian subcontinent	11.4	16.3	14.1
Irish Republic	6.5	2.8	0.7
Other – Europe	3.0	1.2	1
Other – Commonwealth	2.3	3.4	0.54
Other	2.0	2.3	1.8

(Source: GMP Census, October 1996. Unrestricted principals – England and Wales)

Discussion

1 There are currently more than 34 000 GP principals registered in the UK. They form the largest group of senior doctors in the NHS and are an expensive commodity.

2 Female GPs now represent almost 31% of the total workforce in general practice which has clear implications for the future. Only 68% of females are contracted for full-time work compared with 95% of males. What effect is this going to have in terms of future healthcare planning? Should the balance be addressed or would this contravene sex discrimination legislation?

3 The 1990 Contract and the Conservative government White Papers *Primary Care – The Future* and *Choice and Opportunity* provided and planned for more flexible working arrangements in general practice. However, will this lead to fewer GPs being available to provide future care?

4 The number of doctors in England rose by 11% between 1985 and 1995, thereby providing 54.6 GPs per 100 000 population. Has this growth been necessary and what factors have influenced it in the past and are likely to do so in the future?

5 Eighteen percent of GP principals in UK qualified 'overseas'. The NHS would have been undermanned without them in the 1960s and 1970s but how are they going to be replaced in the future and from which nations? Are we likely to have more EEC graduates settling in the UK in the new millennium?

6 The mean list size of GPs had fallen to 1887 in 1995. Is there such a thing as an ideal list size and how should we calculate this mythical figure?

7 The average age of GPs is going down, partly driven by enforced retirement of the over-70s after the 1990 Contract. GPs are retiring at an earlier stage also and are looking for lives beyond medicine. What effects will this have on the provision of care in the future?

8 As we consider the roles of all members of the primary healthcare team, are GP principals required in the same numbers as in the past?

6

The health team

General practice has evolved from single-handed GPs often doing everything themselves and working from barely suitable premises – sometimes their own homes – to a large team with many supporting staff. These include receptionists, computer operators, secretaries, managers, dispensers in dispensing practices, as well as attached staff employed by the local health authority or trust. This latter group may include community midwives, district nurses, health visitors and community psychiatric nurses.

The advent of fundholding in the early 1990s gave GPs much more control over whom they employ. The remuneration in fundholding practices switched from the 70% reimbursement per whole-time equivalent (WTE) to a total staff budget, derived from historical data, which the practice could spend as it saw fit. Other budgets were given for community services, prescribing and hospital referrals. If savings were made in any of these three areas, the money could be used to improve areas of patient care or the premises, subject to approval by the HA. Many practices now employ physiotherapists, complementary therapists and counsellors, for example. Others have increased nursing hours to allow specific strategies to be carried out, for example weight reduction and stop smoking clinics. Budgetary allocations made allowance for the employment of fundholding managers and data collection staff.

Who are the health team?

The health team comprises several groups of workers whose roles should be clearly defined and understood.

General practitioners are the employers and are responsible in law for the actions of their staff, though day-to-day supervision is usually delegated to the practice manager. GPs contract with the HA to provide recognised services and receive reimbursement from the HA for that provision. They are, in the main, unrestricted principals but there are also assistants and registrars (who are employees).

The *practice manager* is responsible for the business and organisational side of the practice. Often they have been promoted from another position within the practice but there are numerous courses to gain the required skills. He or she will usually be familiar with the computer systems in the practice.

Receptionists are the first point of contact with the practice. This may be by phone or in person and it is clearly a vital role. Many practices have introduced protocols to help receptionists to meet patients' and doctors' needs. Some may give simple advice in accordance with these. They are responsible for record filing and distribution and increasingly are required to operate computerised appointment systems.

Secretaries/computer operators may also work in reception or the dispensary in addition to their recording and communication roles.

Practice nurses have become vital to the team in terms of both pure nursing skills and ensuring that targets are met in areas which attract additional remuneration, such as immunisations and cervical cytology. They now do many tasks previously undertaken by the GP and there has been much debate about what is appropriate for nurses to do. It seems likely that with training and accreditation, more *nurse practitioners* with extended roles will appear in the near future.

The attached members, employed by the local health authority or trust, are:

- the *district nurse*, concerned primarily with home visiting to the chronically ill and elderly. They may double as a practice nurse also but have a specific qualification in district nursing which practice nurses do not require
- the *health visitor*, who works predominantly with young families in a role that is mainly supportive and educational in promoting better health
- the *community midwife*, involved in the antenatal and postnatal care of all the maternity cases in the practice
- increasingly, *community psychiatric nurses* and *social workers* are being attached.

Finally, for terminally ill patients it is common to find a *Macmillan nurse* who is a specialist in palliative care. *Marie Curie nurses* and *carers* also play a role with terminally ill patients. Both are funded by charitable foundations and are usually based on a hospital district and cover a number of practices within that area.

How many members?

There has been a steady increase in the numbers of people employed in the health team, particularly because of the additional requirements of data capture and processing associated with fundholding. (There are now nearly 1600 WTE fund managers in England.) There has been a similar rise in the numbers of clerical staff so that there are now two WTE staff members per practitioner compared to 1.1 in 1976 and 1.7 in 1989. Because the vast majority are employed part time the actual numbers are greater, leading to further erosion of the personal touch.

Table 6.1 Analysis of practice staff (England)

Type of staff	Numbers employed – actual	WTEs
Fund manager	2215	1597
Practice manager	8025	6537
Secretarial	10 178	6584
Reception and clerical	48 009	28 764
Computer operator	3412	2269
Other admin	2954	1815
Practice nurse	17 898	9821
Dispenser	1971	1136
Physiotherapist	320	78
Chiropodist	151	29
Interpreter/link worker	172	71
Counsellor	1064	230
Complementary therapist	81	14
Other duties	931	374
Total	97 381	59 319

A practice model

For a practice caring for a population of 10 000 people, the primary care team is likely to comprise the following.

GPs	5 (WTE) Some may be part time or job sharing which would increase numbers
GP staff	
Managers	1–2 (fundholding and ordinary manager)
Receptionists	10 (part time)
Secretaries	2
Practice nurses	3 (part time)
Attached	
District nurses	3
Health visitors	2
Midwives	1 or 2 part time
Others	2 part time
Total	30

Pharmacists

In the UK there are over 12 000 pharmacists in contract with health authorities to supply NHS prescriptions. They are not integral members of the primary care team but, as 33% of the population are self-medicating and another 33% are taking prescribed drugs at any time, many of the population will be in contact with pharmacists. Would it be illogical for them to form closer links with local practices to develop joint general policies on health promotion, disease prevention and management?

Discussion

The NHS has existed for 50 years and in that time general practice has changed profoundly, along with many other facets of life. The norm used to be a single-handed GP caring for approximately 2000–2500 patients, whereas now groups of doctors caring for 10 000 patients within a team of 30–35 attached staff are more common. This has affected all members of the team and patients.

1 Personal care on a one-to-one basis is the core concept of British general practice and is more difficult to achieve in large groups so measures need to be adopted to preserve it.
2 Decision making and management of a large group are complex and the agenda of each individual in the group needs to be given consideration.
3 The internal market imposed by the previous government has heightened awareness that general practice is very much a business and the partners should all be striving to optimise profit. Conflicts of interest arise and can lead to turmoil at all levels, including partners and staff.
4 The role of practice nurses continues to develop. What roles and tasks can be appropriately delegated by GPs?
5 How should attached staff be integrated into the primary healthcare team?
6 Given the communication difficulties highlighted above, what is the optimal size of the PHCT?
7 With one pharmacy per 5000 head of population and with 66% of the population taking medicine daily, how can/should pharmacists be more fully integrated into the PHCT?
8 As PHCT size increases, should GPs be the only partners?
9 Should patients be involved and represented legally in the work and services provided by primary care?

7

Practices

The organisation of practices has changed enormously since 1948, and merging of principals into group partnerships has been the trend over the past 20 years. The number of single-handed GPs has decreased from about 43% in 1952 to 10% in 1995. Likewise, larger practice units have emerged and whereas only 1% of practices had six or more partners in 1952, currently 12% have 6+ partners.

These changes have resulted in GPs sharing facilities, including premises, staff and equipment. This in turn results in economies of scale which allow the provision of better services for patients and enhance GPs' own working conditions by sharing out-of-hours cover, costs and facilities. An added incentive for change was the 1966 Charter which introduced extra remuneration for GPs working in groups of three or more.

The mean partnership size was 1–2 GPs in 1952 and 4–5 in 1990. The number of practices in England and Wales has therefore been reduced in this period and in 1996 there were 9561. In 1996, 2883 GPs were single handed, though some work from premises shared with other practitioners. The number of partnerships by partnership size is shown in Figure 7.1.

Figure 7.1 Number of partnerships by partnership size.

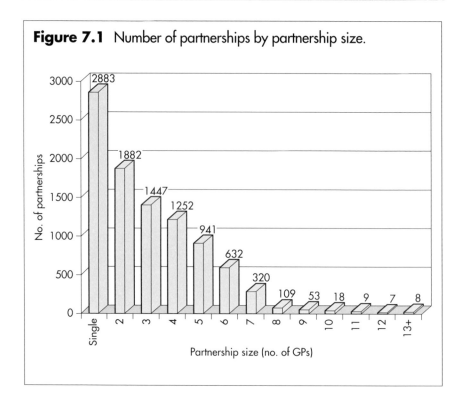

Health centres

A major feature of the 1948 NHS blueprint was the formation of 'health centres', which were purpose-built premises provided and managed by local authorities for rental by GPs. Attractive in theory, they never became popular with GPs, who preferred to develop their own practices suited to their individual/group practice needs. Attractive loans and support from the NHS via the cost-rent scheme allowed many such practices to be built throughout the 1980s and early 1990s, though many authorities are becoming more reluctant to sanction such schemes given the present economic climate.

Fundholding

After the introduction of the GP fundholding scheme in 1990 the number of GP fundholders grew steadily until the election of the Labour government in 1997.

Table 7.1 Number of fundholding practices

	1991	1992	1993	1994	1995	1996	1997	Cumulative 1991–97
UK	326	312	792	957	596	1406	710	2362
England	305	280	659	835	524	1122	513	2079
Wales	7	19	48	43	29	64	23	119
Scotland	14	13	65	55	17	172	137p	120p
N. Ireland	–	–	20	24	26	48	37	44

(Source: OHE Compendium of Health Statistics, 1995) (p = provisional)
Note: In N. Ireland, the fundholding scheme was first introduced in 1993.

Practices have altered their *modus operandi* since the introduction of fundholding and there have been many perceived benefits, including the modification and improvement of practice premises and patient facilities from fund savings.

Commissioning

Commissioning is when GPs form into groups in order to try to exert some influence over health authorities in determining how resources for healthcare are allocated. Originally, this encompassed all aspects of healthcare need, including the planning, purchasing and monitoring of the quality of healthcare. The main difference between commissioning and fundholding was that commissioning groups did not hold their own budgets. Whereas fundholding was recognised by the previous Conservative government, commissioning was not resourced; however, by 1996 the National Association of Commissioning GPs were aware of more than 8000 GPs involved in known commissioning groups.

The Labour government signalled its intent to abolish fundholding in a series of White Papers published in December 1997 and January 1998, the focus of which was the devolution of decision making to a local level. This was done through the formation of primary care groups (PCGs) comprising health professionals led by GPs. Fundholding was abolished in March 1999 and the new groups came into existence in April 1999. In England, each group controls its own budget and has the freedom to make decisions about resource allocation so long as this meets local health targets. The key aims of the PCGs are to develop primary care by joint working across practices, provide a forum for professional development, audit and peer review, and to assure quality in the delivery of care. There are four levels of entry for groups at the outset.

Discussion

1 GPs have chosen to remain as private independent contractors to the NHS and so the change from solo to group practice has been largely self-determined, albeit with external pressures from a succession of government initiatives. Should GPs remain private independent contractors? Does their development need to be more planned locally and/or nationally?

2 The assumption throughout has been that 'bigger is better'. The question that must be asked is 'better for whom?'. Have patients experienced a reduction in personal primary care as a result of management/organisational changes?

3 Clearly there have been advantages for GPs in terms of holiday and out-of-hours co-operation plus regular opportunity for professional discussion and intercourse. Is this the most effective and efficient way of providing this service?

4 What is the optimum size of group practice? How is optimum measured and does it depend on locality? Should research be done in this area before future policies are decided?

5 The gatekeeping role of the GP has been influenced by the fundholding concept. Has this been the most efficient way of producing improvements in secondary care services for patients and at what cost to the GPs? How will commissioning alter this gatekeeping role?

6 Are there collaborative measures with local hospitals that have produced better outcomes for patients? If so, what are we doing to enhance them for the future?

7 How is the formation of primary care groups going to affect the organisation of practices for the future? Is the independent contractor status of GPs in jeopardy? Is salaried service likely to become a chosen career path or may it become the only option?

8

The work

In other chapters we have considered the way in which the primary care team has evolved, as well as the things which have driven these changes. This chapter considers the overall work which the doctor does. This is because, at the time of writing, no data which indicate the work carried out by other members of the team exist in accessible form, which is in itself perhaps a reflection of how rapidly practice has evolved in this decade. The reader should appreciate that the statistics used in these chapters are 2–3 years old in the most part by the time they are compiled.

It should be remembered that these figures provide an objective assessment of quantity only. Quality is very much harder to assess objectively, at both an individual and population level. *Our Healthier Nation* (The Stationery Office, 1998) requires health authorities to promote strategies which will promote an overall health gain for the population, but it fails to define exactly what that gain should be. Similarly, most GPs would balk at trying to define health gain for their practice populations and perhaps congratulate themselves on simply doing no harm!

The volume of work

One of general practice's greatest rewards is its diversity. Thus, in a typical week, a GP may expect to consult in his office and at the patient's home and offer advice or negotiate with patients using the telephone. Some doctors continue to offer intrapartum care both at home and on GP maternity units. Scope exists for interest in a particular field to be furthered by working regular hospital sessions. Non-clinical activity may include patient administration, practice administration, discussion with partners and hospital colleagues, postgraduate education, undergraduate teaching and so on.

Knowledge of the practice population, consultation rates and variables affecting the latter, such as the number of patients over 75, numbers of unemployed, single mothers, etc., allows sufficient consulting time to be planned, so relieving stress in doctors, staff and patients. This perhaps sounds obvious, but relaxed doctors and staff probably provide a higher quality of care and enjoy their work more.

Patient consulting rates

A well-known truism has pertained until recently and was quoted in the previous edition of this book so was accurate then.

- In any year 70% of all persons consult their GP at least once.
- In any year 90% of families consult their GP at least once.
- In five years the GP will treat over 90% of his patients.

Morbidity statistics from the General Practice Fourth National Study (MSGP 4, 1991–92) though, reveal that 78% of patients consult at least once per year and that, as previously, the young and old consult more frequently.

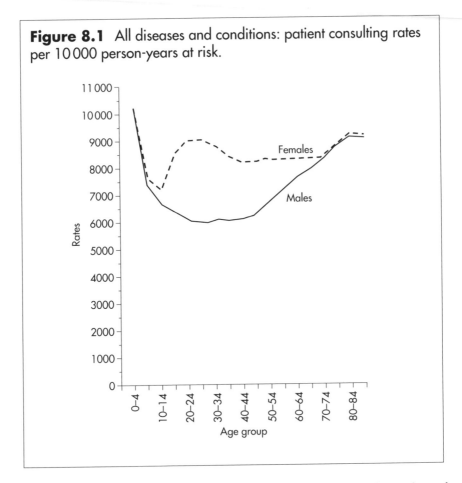

Figure 8.1 All diseases and conditions: patient consulting rates per 10 000 person-years at risk.

The *annual consultation rate (ACR) per patient* is the total number of consultations in the year divided by the number of patients on the doctor's list. So, if there are 8000 consultations in a year in a practice population of 2000, the annual consultation rate per patient is 4.0.

The reported range of consultation rates is under 2 to over 6 and varies according to many factors. The average rate appears to be between 3 and 4. There does seem to have been a reduction over the past few years, as inspection of the MSGP 4 reveals.

Table 8.1 Change in ACR 1950–91

Year	Annual consultation rate
1950–51	3.7
1970–71	3.0
1980–81	3.5
1991–92	2.9

Place of consultation

Whereas in the 1950s and 1960s it would not be unusual for roughly 20% of consultations to be in the patient's home, pressure of time and differing expectations in society today mean that in most practices now the home visiting rate has dropped to between 3% and 5% of the total consultation rate.

Telephone consultations

Historically these were not a large feature of British general practice though there is some evidence emerging that this is a more common method of doctor–patient contact. Anecdotally it would appear that this may have developed because of the increasing numbers of out-of-hours co-ops. The emphasis on patients travelling to a care centre after hours rather than the GP doing the traditional home visit seems to have led to (and still be leading to) improved negotiation about where the most appropriate place for the consultation is. Additionally, alterations in GP terms of service in 1995 allowed doctors to dictate the most appropriate place for any consultation. Given the increasing tendency toward 'charterism', it may be prudent for practitioners to consider screening visit requests on the telephone prior to agreeing to the visits. This, of course, must be balanced against the increasing incidence of litigation.

Out-of-hours cover

There is huge variation in the demands made on GPs by patients out of hours, depending on such factors as urban/rural population, socioeconomic class, cultural differences, and availability of alternative advice from friends and family. There is also evidence that systems within practices affecting the availability of appointments are equally important.

Notwithstanding these factors, in the last decade there has been a marked rise in the demands made by patients out of hours, which is probably a result of many factors. GPs have responded by increased use of deputising services and the formation of GP out-of-hours co-operatives in which a number of practices within a given area band together to offer cover to each other's patients out of hours. These co-ops operate from a (roughly) central location and usually employ drivers and have fairly sophisticated message-answering systems. Table 8.2 shows that GPs typically use more than one arrangement for covering the out-of-hours period. Over half of all GPs use a co-operative and 30% use a deputising service at least part of the time.

Table 8.2 GPs' out-of-hours arrangements

Type of arrangement	Percentage of all GPs
Own	57
Local arrangement	17.2
Co-operative	51.2
Deputising service	29.9

Table 8.3 Number of hours typically spent on call each week

Type of arrangement	Average per GP (hours)
Own	26.8
Local arrangement	18.9
Co-operative	5.5

The data in Table 8.4 are from a co-op which was established in February 1996 based in a rural Lincolnshire market town. The co-op comprises 24 principals.

Table 8.4 GP co-operative data March 1998

Total population	47 363
No. of patient contacts	530
Contacts /1000 patients	11.19
No. of home visits	127
% home visits	24%
No. of telephone advice	277
% telephone advice	52%
No. seen at centre	126
% seen at centre	24%
No. sent to A&E unseen	49
Total no. admitted	44
No. of night visits	55
Night visits/1000 population	1.16

Undoubtedly there will be a great deal of variation between co-ops but anecdotally their introduction does appear to be lessening the out-of-hours demand and, although initially patients appeared to resist, there has been gradual acceptance.

At the time of writing, data pertaining to the number of GPs in co-ops and those using deputising services are not available.

Time distribution

Patient contact now appears to account for 70% of a GP's time and this is reflected by the findings shown in Table 8.5. The same source estimates that, excluding on-call duties, GPs work just over 39 hours per week (39.21) and expresses surprise, as the perception amongst GPs is that work volumes had increased. Direct comparison with previous data is not possible as like-for-like data were not collected.

Table 8.5 Time spent by GPs on different activities

Activity	% of time spent on activity in normal working hours
Patient contact	70
Patient administration	13
Practice administration	8
Other GMS work	6
Non-GMS work	3

(Source: Review Body on Doctors' and Dentists' Remuneration (27th report), 1998)

Table 8.6 Comparison of surgery and consultation times 1990–97

Activity	1990	1997
Average no. of surgery sessions per week	8.47	8.38
Average length of surgery sessions	2h 22m	2h 44m
Average length of consultations	8.33m	9.36m

(Source: Review Body on Doctors' and Dentists' Remuneration (27th report), 1998)

Discussion

1 Workload of GPs is a highly sensitive subject. Whilst quantity is relatively easy to measure, quality is much more difficult to assess.

2 There is a large variation in mean annual consultation rates. Why are there differences and can/should these be addressed?

3 The number and proportion of home visits has decreased. Is this addressing the needs of the doctors or the patients?

4 The number of night visits has doubled over the past ten years and this has been in part responsible for the introduction of co-operative and commercial deputising services. Is it realistic in the face of this demand to expect GPs to provide 24-hour cover for patients from 'cradle to grave'?

9

Prescribing

It is appropriate to start this chapter with some housekeeping information regarding data and definitions.

The data used in the preparation of this chapter relate to items actually *dispensed*, either by a pharmacist, a dispensing doctor or appliance supplier. They were obtained via the Prescription Pricing Authority (PPA) which processes all prescriptions that are dispensed. There is no consideration given here to items *prescribed* by a doctor but not dispensed because the patient fails to present the prescription for processing. That is in itself worthy of comment but is not considered relevant in the context of this book.

The terms 'prescription' and 'item' are not synonymous. In Department of Health statistics a prescription refers to the form on which the GP has prescribed. This may contain one or several items.

Medicine taking is a very common human activity and a study in 1976 revealed that roughly 66% of the world's population is taking medication of some kind at any given point in time. This divides roughly into 50% taking prescribed medication and 50% taking medicine bought over the counter (OTC).

In the UK the majority of prescribing costs are met by the NHS and the following is a consideration of various aspects of the effect of prescribing.

How much prescribing?

The amount of prescribing has increased progressively in the UK (and elsewhere!) over the past 40 years so that the number of prescribed items per capita are as shown in Table 9.1.

Table 9.1 Number of prescription items per capita

	1960	1970	1980	1990	1993
Annual prescriptions per person	4.7	5.5	6.6	7.7	8.8

(Source: OHE Compendium of Health Statistics, 1995)

In all, the number of prescriptions (items) dispensed has grown from 225 million in 1949 to 512 million in 1993, corresponding to a rise from 4.5 to 8.8 items per person.

There is a wide variation in prescribing rates between GPs in the four nations of the UK; the rates per capita in Wales and Northern Ireland are always higher than in Scotland and England by approximately one-fifth. In England generally, a high frequency and rate of rise of prescribing has been seen in the north and north western parts of the country where levels of morbidity and unemployment are correspondingly greater.

As seen in the previous chapter, where it was noted that the elderly generated a greater than average amount of work, so they generate a greater number of prescriptions as is shown in Table 9.2. There undoubtedly has been an increase in total numbers of elderly people but even on a per capita basis it can be seen that their prescribing requirements have increased.

Table 9.2 Prescription items per person by age group (England)

Year	Elderly*	Under 16**	Chargeable
1990	17.4	4.2	2.7
1991	18.0	4.3	2.4
1992	18.9	4.4	2.3
1993	19.8	4.8	2.2

*Elderly: men 65 and over; women 60 and over.
**Children under 16 and people aged under 19 in full-time education.

What for?

Medicine is prone to follow trends which are dictated largely by the development of new drugs as well as the emergence of data collected and publicised about older drugs. The influence of the media, the public and marketing by pharmaceutical companies should be borne in mind also. Thus sedatives and tranquillisers (mainly benzodiazepines), which were the most commonly prescribed drugs in 1978, had slipped to the seventh most commonly prescribed drugs in 1988 behind such things as new cardiovascular preparations (ACE inhibitors, calcium antagonists and beta-blockers) and antiasthmatics (Action Asthma campaign since the early 1980s) (*see* Table 9.3).

Regulation of new drugs

Each year in the UK approximately 600 new licences for pharmaceutical products are granted. Of these, 5–10% are for completely new preparations (new active substance or NAS) and the rest are for established products in new doses, formulations or combinations. Each NAS costs the industry about £100 million to research and develop and the company has a 20-year patent to recoup that cost. Thereafter other companies can produce the same drug.

Table 9.3 The most commonly prescribed drugs: 1978, 1988 and 1995

	1978	1988	1995
1	Sedatives and tranquillisers	CVS preparations	CNS preparations
2	Minor analgesics	Dermatological preparations	CVS preparations
3	Dermatological preparations	Anti-asthma drugs	Anti-infective preparations
4	Penicillins	Diuretics	Respiratory drugs
5	Diuretics	Penicillins	Gastrointestinal drugs
6	Cough medicines	Minor analgesics	Dermatological preparations
7	CVS preparations	Anti-inflammatory preparations	Musculoskeletal preparations
8	Hypnotics	Hypnotics	
9	Anti-inflammatory preparations	Sedatives and tranquillisers	
10	Anti-asthma drugs	Other anti-infective drugs	

The system of classification unfortunately changed between 1988 and 1995.

The *Medicines Act 1968* provides the legal regulatory framework governing the supply and use of medicines in the UK. The Medicines Control Agency (MCA) administers the act. It overseas the manufacture, promotion and distribution of medicines and can inspect factories in the UK and abroad to check for purity of ingredients. Product licences, which must be held for a drug to be sold in the UK, are granted by the MCA. The MCA grants a licence if it feels that a product is safe and effective and can give overall benefit.

The Committee on Safety of Medicines (CSM) was set up by the Medicines Commission which advises ministers on implementation of the Medicines Act. The CSM advises on questions of efficacy, safety and quality of new medicines.

PACT data

Since August 1994, a PACT standard report has been issued to every practising GP on a three-monthly basis. The report contains prescribing costs and rates of the practice compared with the local and national patterns and with practice data from previous years. These are broken down further into the top six therapeutic groups of the BNF, the leading 20 drugs prescribed by the practice together with the proportion of new medicines prescribed. The availability of drugs where generic prescribing would reduce cost is also indicated.

PACT data recognise that elderly patients generally require more prescriptions than patients in other age groups. Thus, for comparative purposes the patient population is described in terms of prescribing units or PUs. Under the system, patients aged 65 and over count as three PUs on the basis that they require on average three times as many prescriptions as the under–65s.

Selected list

Since 1 April 1985 the government's selected list has curtailed the range of drugs available for prescription on the NHS in certain therapeutic categories; drugs included on the list cannot be prescribed on the NHS. An extended limited list was announced in November 1992 to include a further ten therapeutic categories containing about 1500 preparations in total. As yet, decisions have only been taken in five of the ten categories and an extra 63 preparations have been blacklisted. If patients require drugs on the list they have to pay the full cost of the drug via private prescription.

Costs

The NHS drug bill has always accounted for approximately 10% of the total NHS budget. It was over £3 million in 1992 and had risen to £3.6 million in 1993. This is reflected in the per capita figures in Table 9.4.

Table 9.4 Total cost of NHS prescriptions expressed per capita (UK)

Year	1984	1986	1988	1990	1992	1994	1996
Per capita cost (£)	31	36	44	52	64	74	87
Per Rx (£)	4.4	5.1	5.9	6.7	7.6	8.3	9.1

In case it is thought that the annual UK cost of drugs per capita is exceptionally high, comparisons with other countries shows otherwise (*see* Table 9.5).

Table 9.5 Per capita expenditure on drugs (£) 1992

Country	Expenditure per capita (£)
Japan	168
Germany	163
USA	157
France	139
Italy	128
Luxembourg	115
Belgium	114
Canada	88
Spain	83
Portugal	78
Denmark	73
UK	68
Netherlands	66
Ireland	63
Greece	37

The number of items issued per person is also less than in other European countries.

Figure 9.1 Drug expenditure per capita by country.

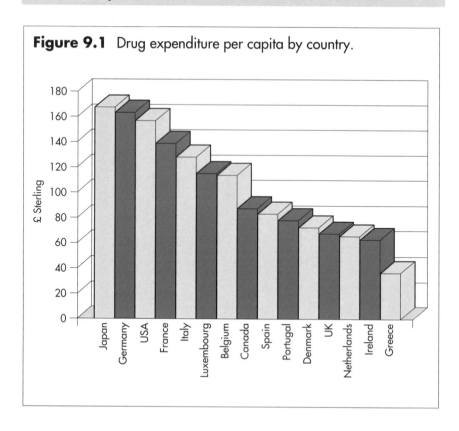

Table 9.6 Numbers of items prescribed, by country

Country	Year	Number
Italy	1990	21.1
Austria	1989	17.0
Portugal	1989	16.5
France	1992	16.0
Spain	1989	14.8
Germany	1989	12.0
Belgium	1989	9.3
UK	1993	8.8
Switzerland	1989	7.5
Denmark	1990	5.9

Self-medication

OTC medication is bought over the counter either at a pharmacist or other medicines outlet, such as supermarkets and garage forecourts. It requires no prescription or previous medical advice, though many doctors now are advising patients to self-medicate on the grounds of cost (simple medications are often cheaper than paying prescription charges) and the greater number of remedies licensed for OTC supply.

The most frequent symptoms for which self-medication is undertaken are:

tiredness	35%
headaches	30%
non-specific aches and pains	25%
overweight	20%
backache	15%
other	30%

The value of these sales is significant as Table 9.7 shows.

Table 9.7 Value of OTC sales

	1996 £m	1997 £m	Growth %
OTC market	1257.8	1349.6	7.3

(Source: MS OTCPlus/PAGP industry estimates)

The breakdown of the shares of sales enjoyed by each group of remedies is given in Table 9.8.

Table 9.8 Market share and growth, by remedy

Group	Share %	Growth % (over previous year)
Pain relievers	16.0	5.3
Skin treatments	12.2	6.6
Cold remedies	8.0	0.5
Sore throat remedies	7.68	4.8
Cough remedies	5.4	4.5
Food supplements	9.4	3.5
Indigestion remedies	5.1	7.5
Oral hygiene	4.6	11.7
Vitamins and minerals	6.7	4.5
Smoking cessation	2.5	11.0
Eye care	1.6	4.4
Hay fever remedies	2.1	2.1
Laxatives	1.8	5.0
Topical pain relievers	2.3	11.0
Acne treatments	1.6	10.6
Antidiarrhoeals	1.8	6.6
Stomach upset remedies	1.4	5.8
Sleeping and calming	0.9	6.0
Antihaemorrhoids	0.8	6.0
Gynaecological products	1.2	13.5
Ear care	0.4	7.0
Cystitis treatments	0.3	3.0
Travel sickness	0.3	−2.5
Worm treatments	0.1	−2.5
Others	5.9	9.0
Total cost	£1349.6 million	

(Source: PAGB Annual Report, 1998)

Discussion

1 GPs write prescriptions in 65% of consultations. What factors might influence this?

2 How can the effectiveness of this level of prescribing be measured and would doing so threaten the independent status of GPs?

3 The levels of prescribing of different drugs can be affected not only by new drug developments but also by trends within society and the NHS in particular, e.g. the change in hospital discharge rates has meant that GPs now have prescribing costs for drugs previously prescribed by hospital practitioners.

4 The volume of prescribing has increased. There are now 8.8 items prescribed per person per year at an annual per capita cost of £68. This has occured because GPs are treating conditions previously dealt with in hospital and also treating conditions which were previously untreatable.

5 Approximately 50% of GP prescriptions are repeats or for unseen patients. How appropriate is this?

6 The most expensive drugs are those for cardiac, rheumatic and GI conditions while the cheapest are analgesics, skin and eye preparations.

7 Per capita costs for prescribed drugs are less in the UK than in many comparable countries. Given this fact, is it appropriate for government via health authorities to be introducing measures to reduce costs further?

10

GPs and hospitals

Healthcare involves co-operation and collaboration between specialists in primary care (GPs) and specialists within secondary care, who are usually based in hospitals. Since the advent of fundholding in the early 1990s, however, some specialists in secondary care have contracted to do outpatient clinics either at the GPs, premises or at small community hospitals or health centres. This move is popular with patients but may not make best use of the hospital specialists' time.

Hospital utilisation

Only 5–10% of consultations in general practice lead to hospital referral but the overall use of hospitals is greater than this. In spite of steadily increasing utilisation of hospitals over the past four decades, the number of inpatient beds has declined so that nationally there are now less than three acute beds per 1000 population and in a few areas this figure is less than two (source: OHE Compendium of Health Statistics, 1995).

Table 10.1 Hospital utilisation rates 1949–95

Per 1000 population	1949	1959	1969	1979	1989	1995
Hospital beds	10.3	10.3	9.5	8.0	6.5	4.9
Inpatients	67	88	109	117	139	
New outpatient referrals	140	159	166	167	177	
A&E attendances	89	121	166	198	231	

This has been achieved by shorter inpatient stays for given procedures and a shift of resources from secondary care to the community. In spite of a number of innovative schemes to support the early transfer of inpatients to their homes, many practitioners still doubt the wisdom of such moves and argue that without greater resources than are currently available, patient care will be compromised. Political considerations and the confidence of GPs to care for recently acutely ill patients need to be taken into account.

Domiciliary consultations

These are reducing in number generally with the exception of consultations for elderly and psychiatric cases. Whilst originally designed to be a joint consultation between patient, GP and specialist, in reality a specialist usually visits alone.

GPs in hospitals

There are two ways in which GPs can be involved in hospital work:

- in community hospitals
- in district general hospitals.

They operate as clinical assistants and as hospital practitioners.

Table 10.2 GP appointments in hospitals 1986–96 (England)

Year	1986		1996	
	Number	WTE	Number	WTE
Hospital practitioners	850	210	810	180
Clinical assistants	6870	1840	5940	1790

This shows a 14% reduction (WTE) in the number of hospital practitioners and a 3% reduction (WTE) in the number of clinical assistants over the ten-year period.

Unfortunately, because of a change in the method of compilation of statistics since the previous version of this book was published, it is not possible to obtain figures for the number of cottage hospitals in existence.

Discussion

1 There has been a massive swing from secondary (hospital-based) care towards care in the community. Has sufficient been done in terms of resources, training and finances to ensure that this care is effectively and efficiently delivered?

2 Five to ten percent of consultations result in referral to hospital. In one year, 14% of the practice population will be admitted one or more times. Eighteen percent are newly referred to outpatient departments and 23% attend accident and emergency departments.

3 The number of GP hospital appointments appears to be declining. Why is that happening and what will be the effect on levels of skill in given specialities in primary care?

11

Female doctors

The NHS is still the largest employer of women in the UK. Over 75% of its employees are female and they make up 31% of all practitioners engaged in general practice. The proportion of female GPs continues to increase and medical schools are now producing more female than male graduates. Additionally, female graduates are more likely to choose a career in general practice than their male counterparts.

GP principals

In 1950, less than 10% of GP principals were female; in 1996, 29% were female and there has been a steady increase as shown in Table 11.1.

Table 11.1 Percentage of female GP principals

1950	1970	1980	1985	1986	1987	1988	1989	1990	1996
<10	10	17	19	20	21	22	23	24	29

(Source: GMS Statistics England and Wales, 1996)

However, 31% of all GP practitioners are now female if assistants and registrars are included and 54% of all registrars are currently female.

Contractual commitment of female GPs

The average list sizes of female GPs have traditionally been smaller than those of men and in 1996, average list sizes had fallen overall to 1882 in England and 1719 in Wales. Additionally, 95.3% of male GPs had full-time contractual obligations whereas only 68.4% of female GPs were working full time.

Examinations

It is worth remarking that female registrars do better in the MRCGP examination than their male counterparts, with the pass rate for females being 86.5% and for males 73.9%.

Table 11.2 MRCGP pass rates

	Sat MRCGP	Passed MRCGP	%
Male	696	515	73.9
Female	736	637	86.5

(Source: RCGP Members' Reference Book, 1996)

Career problems for female GPs

Female GPs report many obvious problems when interviewed about their careers, which include:

- having to give priority to their husband's careers (often medical)
- pressures and stresses of domestic and family duties
- interruptions to and difficulties with attempting to carry out full-time postgraduate vocational training
- partners presenting problems regarding maternity leave
- finding suitably flexible employment to combine professional and domestic aspirations.

Parkhouse (1991)* produced detailed reports on problems encountered by female GPs. His extensive research showed that whilst general practice was the first career choice of new medical graduates, ten years after graduation only 61% of females had become GP principals (64% with no break in training) whereas 90% of male graduates had principalship (96% without training breaks).

Of social interest was the fact that more male GPs were married and had children than their female counterparts but of the female GPs with no children, 83% were working full time. Parenthood clearly has an effect on female careers in general practice: 40% of childless women GPs had experienced a period of unemployment, 63% of female GPs with one or two children had been unemployed and 77% of female GPs with three or more children had suffered this difficulty.

With increasing numbers of females graduating and entering general practice, it is clear that the government and the profession must identify and deal with the problems outlined above. More flexible career choices since 1990 have improved the options for the female GP cadre but much more attention is required if one considers the fact that in future, it is likely that 50% or more of GP principals will be female.

* Parkhouse J (1991) *Doctor's Careers.* Routledge, London.

Discussion

1 The number and proportion of female GP principals continue to increase and this needs to be taken into account by both the profession and the government in order to plan for future health needs. Should the likelihood of >50% of GP principals being female be allowed to become reality?
2 Flexible career options need to be made available to the female GP cadre to prevent periods of employment difficulty and to allow professional and domestic integration. Are part-time jobs or job sharing the best options available?
3 Should the option of artificially increasing the proportion of male medical graduates be addressed or explored?
4 Will the increasing trend towards salaried service provide more suitable career options for female GPs?

12

Education and training

There are many stages that are recognised in the education process of a GP but for the purposes of this book we will consider under three broad categories:

- undergraduate – where medical students are given a brief introduction to general practice
- general practice vocational training (GPVT) – currently lasts for three years and has been mandatory for NHS GP principals since 1982
- continuing medical education – traditionally a responsibility of GPs.

Undergraduate

The General Medical Council has stated that all UK medical schools should include some teaching on general practice in their curricula and this recommendation has been universally adopted. All UK medical schools now have departments of general practice, though the length of time spent on such courses and the emphasis placed on general practice by the different schools vary enormously.

Selection procedures vary between medical schools and are not particularly geared towards producing a particular type of doctor. Approximately 10% of medical students do not complete their training and register within the five-year allotted period. The cost of training a medical student is over £300 000.

General Medical Council (GMC) registrations

Table 12.1 shows the pattern of full, provisional and limited registration over the past five years with the GMC. It also demonstrates for the same period the granting of full registration to practitioners from member states of the European Economic Area (EEA).

Since 10 June 1977 the GMC has been required to grant full registration to nationals of member states of the European Union (EU) who hold qualifications granted in a member state. Since 1 January 1994 European Community provisions on the mutual recognition of doctors' qualifications have also applied to Iceland and Norway which, together with the EU member states, constitute the EEA.

Table 12.1 GMC registration

	1993	1994	1995	1996	1997
UK, provisional	3685	3697	3840	3961	4030
UK, full	3675	3657	3710	3822	3920
Overseas, provisional	252	254	324	504	402
Overseas, full	2500	2539	3327	4047	3678
EEA, full	1188	1444	1779	2084	1860
Total for all areas of qualification					
Provisional	3937	3951	4164	4465	4432
Full	7363	7640	8816	9953	9458

Vocational training

The number of GP trainees/registrars increased twofold from 1976 to 1989 but now averages approximately 1700/year. This means that there are 5100 registrars on a three-year scheme at any one time in the UK. At present, the majority of schemes allow only 12 months in the general practice setting, though this looks likely to change in the foreseeable future. The Armed Services have always provided 18 months training in general practice and 18 months in hospital posts.

The GPVT scheme is under the supervision of the Joint Committee for Postgraduate Training in General Practice (JCPTGP) and this committee issues certificates of satisfactory completion of the prescribed course or for an equivalent programme. There has been much criticism of the lack of objectivity in this system in the past and, partly as a result of this and a wish to raise the standard of GPs entering the profession as principals, the JCPTGP has introduced a process of summative assessment along with a more structured approach to GP principal approval. Summative assessment became mandatory with the changes to the Vocational Training Regulations in September 1997. The JCPTGP will remain responsible for issuing certificates and has made a commitment that these certificates should continue to reflect current thinking in the general practice branch of the profession. A great deal of work and effort went into the development of more structured assessment of registrars in 1995–96 and it is hoped that the gap which existed for years, which allowed 75–100 doctors to enter the profession who needed more education, will soon be closed.

Table 12.2 Approved trainers

	1990	1991	1992	1993	1994	1995	1996	1997
England	2726	2824	2940	3015	3108	3195	3216	3292
Wales	275	268	264	265	267	264	259	256
Scotland	350	354	357	358	353	368	365	341
Gt. Britain	3351	3446	3561	3638	3728	3827	3840	3889

(Source: DoH. N. Ireland Office was only able to supply registrar statistics)

Approximately one-third of practices are now recognised for GPVT and 11% of GPs in England are trainers.

In future, registrars wishing to become registered as principals will be required to pass summative assessment, obtain a satisfactory extended report from their trainer (signed VTR1), be able to demonstrate satisfactory consulting skills by video assessment and have produced a satisfactory audit/project.

Table 12.3 GP registrars

	1990	1991	1992	1993	1994	1995	1996	1997
England	1562	1639	1613	1529	1445	1404	1305	1343
Wales	148	138	133	124	118	104	66	95
Scotland	330	325	321	303	278	282	234	240
Gt Britain	2040	2102	2067	1956	1841	1790	1605	1678
N. Ireland	56	45	46	45	45	45	48	40
UK	2096	2147	2113	2001	1886	1835	1653	1718

(Source: DoH)

JCPTGP

The JCPTGP has been issuing certificates since 1981. Over the subsequent 14 years 31 522 certificates were issued and 174 refused, which represents only 0.55%. Of the certificates issued, 26 636 were for prescribed courses and 4886 for equivalents (to prescribed experience).

Table 12.4 JCPTGP certificates issued

Year	Prescribed	Equivalent	Ratio P:E	Male	Female	Ratio M:F	Total
1981	2376	186	93:07	1552	1010	61:39	2562
1982	2083	350	86:14	1512	921	62:38	2433
1983	1426	290	83:17	1171	545	68:32	1716
1984	1415	457	76:24	1221	651	65:35	1872
1985	1518	523	74:26	1341	700	66:34	2041
1986	1835	361	84:16	1354	842	62:38	2196
1987	2014	223	90:10	1341	896	60:40	2237
1988	1935	263	88:12	1319	879	60:40	2198
1989	1983	203	91:09	1256	930	58:42	2186
1990	1895	217	90:10	1147	965	54:46	2112
1991	1815	313	85:15	1169	959	55:45	2128
1992	1743	373	82:18	1111	1005	52:48	2116
1993	1556	379	80:20	1029	906	53:47	1935
1994	1564	369	80:20	983	950	51:49	1933
1995	1478	379	79:21	876	981	47:53	1857
Total	26 636	4886					31 522

For certificates granted in 1995, 84.8% were to UK graduates, 6.9% were to overseas graduates and 8.2% to EEC graduates. The fall below 2000 certificates per year since 1992 represents a worrying trend, as there has been disillusionment with the general practice option amongst principals (post-1990 Contract) which is being reflected in the numbers of graduates wishing to pursue a career in general practice.

Royal College of General Practitioners

The total College membership was 17 700 in October 1995, of which 1550 were fellows, 14 771 were members and 1379 were associates. 1049 were from overseas and 5879 were female (33.2%). The route to membership is via examination and 1980 candidates sat the examination in 1995, of whom 1490 passed (75.25%). The vast majority of candidates continue to be registrars at the end of their GPVT schemes.

The pass rates differ by gender, country of birth and place of primary medical education (PME) as shown in Tables 12.5 and 12.6.

Table 12.5 Pass rates to gender

	Sat MRCGP	Passed MRCGP	%
Male	696	515	73.9
Female	736	637	86.5

(Source: RCGP Members' Reference Book, 1996)

Table 12.6 Pass rates by country of birth and PME

	Sat MRCGP	Passed MRCGP	%
Born UK/Eire	1557	1288	82.7
Born overseas	405	201	49.6
PME in UK/Eire	1759	1429	81.2
PME overseas	203	60	29.6
Born and PME in UK/Eire	1550	1285	82.9
Born overseas but PME in UK/Eire	209	144	68.9
Born and PME overseas	196	57	29.1

(Source: RCGP Members' Reference Book, 1996)

Continuing medical education

Since 1991 each GP has been entitled under the 1990 Contract to spend up to £2000 each year on approved education. The Postgraduate Education Allowance (PGEA) has been reimbursable by the NHS. With over 34 000 GP principals in the UK, this represents a bill of over £60 million to buy education. There is evidence that this is not necessarily being used in the most appropriate way and it is likely that CME will become more formalised and possibly linked to recertification or reaccreditation in the future.

Discussion

1   All medical students receive some training in general practice at medical school. How much time should be dedicated to a subject that will involve the careers of the majority of them?

2   Vocational training currently takes three years but is it being delivered in the correct format or combination? Who gains most, the registrars themselves or their employers? Should more audit of this area be undertaken? It currently accounts for just approximately 5500 GP registrars at any one time.

3   Only just over 0.5% of applicants failed to receive certificates of prescribed or equivalent experience from the JCPTGP in the past. Will the introduction of summative assessment and the other more formalised criteria improve the standard at entry to principalship and what will happen to those who do not achieve the required standard?

4   Should registrars be tested for minimal competence or should the MRCGP examination be the standard required for entry into principalship?

5   CME costs in excess of £60 million per year. Is it being delivered appropriately to the needs of the individual, the profession or the government? If not, how could this be done more effectively?

6   With general practice being the largest 'speciality' for new medical graduates, how can we ensure that their standards of training, education and welfare are protected within the restraints of an increasing financial commitment?

13

Practice finance

It would be fair to say that prior to 1990 many GPs had little thought for the financial consequences of their decisions and were content to concentrate on clinical management of their patients and running their practices smoothly.

The introduction of the 1990 Contract and the *Community Care Act 1991* led to a change in the emphasis in primary care or at least a change in GPs' awareness of the financial aspects of their work, apart from that directly connected with remuneration. The objectives of these pieces of legislation were:

- better value for money through efficiency measures and market economy policies
- better services and quality of care for patients through audits and other checks
- health promotion and disease prevention were given greater weight than previously.

These objectives were to be realised through a number of measures, including:

- new financial incentives
- resource management and indicative budgets for prescribing
- the introduction of GP fundholding practices
- improved practice management with promotion of computerisation (again well remunerated), annual reports, audit and teamwork
- encouragement of continuing medical education through payment of a Postgraduate Education Allowance (PGEA)
- continuation of the reimbursements for employed staff and various other costs.

In order to facilitate the change in emphasis which the Act and Contract engendered, item of service payments were introduced as follows:

- screening and medical check-ups for new patients, three-year non-attenders and patients over 75
- child health surveillance
- meeting targets for childhood immunisations and cervical cytology
- health promotion clinics (weight loss, stop smoking, diabetes, etc.)
- minor surgery
- deprivation allowances
- fees for student attachments.

Table 13.1 Cost of NHS general medical services

Year	Cost of GMS £m	GMS as % of NHS cost
1949	776	10.1
1959	887	10.0
1969	1251	8.3
1979	1409	6.2
1989	2448	7.7
1995	3325	8.5
1996	3570	8.9

(Source: OHE Compendium of Health Statistics, 1997)

GP income and expenditure

In determining a GP's reimbursement, the Doctors' and Dentists' Pay Review Body considers a wide range of factors and comes to a gross figure, which includes expenses in running the practice, and a net figure, the intended net annual remuneration (INAR).

GP *income* recommended by the Doctors' and Dentists' Pay Review Body for 1998–99 was £71 903 gross, £49 030 (balancing item £527). The recommended *expenditure* is thus £23 400, comprising staff salaries and wages, supplies, premises, car travel, net capital allowance and other miscellaneous costs.

Table 13.2 GP pay awards 1986–98

	Net pay £	Expenses £	Gross pay £
1986	25 080	11 600	36 591
1988	28 800	13 480	42 219
1990	33 280	14 473	48 023
1992	40 010	20 000	59 977
1994	41 830	22 500	64 031
1996	44 483	23 000	66 998
1998	49 030	23 400	71 903

Table 13.3 Recommended fees for 1998–99 (£)

● Basic practice allowance	7776
● Seniority and deprivation allowances	Variable
● Standard capitation fees	
1 under 65-year-olds	16.65
2 65–74-year-olds	21.95
3 over 75-year-olds	42.50
● Child health surveillance	12.05
● New patient registration	7.35
● Night visits: annual allowance	2245
fee per visit	22.45
● Childhood immunisation (higher rate)	2430
● Pre-school boosters (higher rate)	720
● Cervical cytology (higher rate)	2700
● Other vaccination/immunisation	5.85
● Ordinary contraceptive fee	15.45
● Family planning (IUCD)	51.60
● Health promotion (band 3)	2340
● Chronic disease management: diabetes and asthma, each	410
● Minor surgery per quarter	121
● PGEA	2445
● Maternity services (full)	193
● Training	5325

Table 13.4 Average cost of consultations

	Cost £	Per person (per year) £
1986–87	8.37	37
1989–90	9.88	49
1992–93	14.37	70
1994–95	15.49	73

(Source: OHE Compendium of Health Statistics, 1997)

Table 13.4 demonstrates that at an average cost of £15 per consultation, the total cost for a patient's annual surgery visits amounted to £73 in 1994–95. This is a 97% increase per person in the annual cost of general practice consultations since 1986–87.

14

The future

The past 50 years have seen three major changes in general practice.

- 1948 – the NHS was established.
- 1966 – General Practice Charter.
- 1990 – New Contract.

Each of these changes caused a major rethink of how general practice is carried out and the delivery of the service. Each has had a major effect on doctors' attitudes and, as in life, the changes have been:

- embraced wholeheartedly by some
- resisted by many
- ignored by others.

If the NHS is to function effectively into the millennium it must have access to up-to-date facts and information upon which to base efficiency measures and economic forecasting. The data must be accurate and reliable, meaningful and practical, applicable and collectable, and in a format that can be used throughout the whole of the NHS at all levels. They need to be reviewed regularly, analysed as to their usefulness and disseminated appropriately.

National data

These should include the following.

Demographic data

- Population size and distribution
- Age/sex data – particular attention to <16-year-olds and >65-year-olds as shown throughout this book
- Population trends – birth, fertility and death rates

Health indices

- Life expectancy
- Infant mortality
- Maternal mortality
- Death rates and causes of death
- Preventable deaths
- Morbidity data
- Smoking rates
- Rates of morbidity caused by poverty/deprivation

Economics

- Cost of healthcare
- Sources of funding for health
- Data regarding distribution of costs between general practice, community trusts and hospitals

Resources

- Medical, nursing and other health service manpower
- Numbers of medical students, percentage graduating and percentage leaving the profession
- Distribution of doctors in GP and hospital settings
- Unemployment among doctors
- Community care facilities available
- Hospital facilities/bed numbers

Quality issues

- Satisfaction statistics
- Complaints
- Outcomes of care
- Utilisation rates for available facilities
- Disability rates

Health authority data

Data collection has improved significantly and perhaps more appropriately since the introduction of the purchaser/provider split brought about by fundholding. However, it is important that it is used effectively to predict future needs by paying particular attention to:

- utilisation of services and resources
- costs, expenditure and cost:benefit ratios
- quality of care and outcome measures
- appropriate use of monies available.

The data collected must be in a format that suits both GPs and hospitals so that time can be saved in data transfer/collation.

General practice data

A great deal of emphasis has been put on GP computerisation but there are still myriad systems in use and no 'master plan' as to the sort of data capture that is considered essential or even desirable. Much of the organisation is left to local initiatives and often relies upon the enthusiasm of a few who are not sufficiently powerful to influence national programmes. GP data should certainly address planning and organisation of practice requirements in efficient, effective and economic contexts.

In the last version of this book, the late John Fry called for a nationally agreed set of basic data which should be produced and adapted to be used in all practices. These should include:

- GP practice population by age/sex
- staff – numbers and workload in particular
- work – volume, nature and outcome
- income, expenditure, costs and profits
- specifics – prescribing, referral, hospital service utilisation data
- premises and equipment.

The authors would endorse the previous request and urge political intervention towards this goal which is long overdue.

The future

The information revolution has arrived, as has the 'value for money' ethos of modern-day medical practice. The effect is likely to be a significant shift of the current balance of medical care towards the primary sector. The spectrum of disease has changed, as has its management; additionally, patient expectations have increased exponentially. Now is the time to organise appropriate data collection and analysis so that suitable provision can be made for the future health needs of the most important people of all – our patients.

Discussion

1 Without knowing who does what best, teamwork and delegation of appropriate tasks cannot occur.
2 How can we plan for the future without projections of what we will be required to do, how often and how long it will take?
3 Unless we know the nature and content of our work accurately, how can we manage service provision effectively and implement appropriate change?
4 How can we decide upon appropriate utilisation of finances unless outcomes of GP/hospital/community care are audited to determine effectiveness?
5 Are satisfaction/complaint surveys important or necessary?

Index